Seniors with Age-Related Memory Decline: A Caregiver's Guide

Copyright Page

TITLE: Seniors with Age-Related Memory Decline: A Caregiver's Guide

1ST Edition

ISBN: 9798223524151

Table of Contents

Seniors with Age-Related Memory Decline: A Caregiver's Guide

By Roberto Miguel Rodriguez

Chapter 1: Understanding Age-Related Memory Decline

The Aging Brain: How Memory Changes with Age

As caregivers, it is essential to understand how memory changes with age in order to provide the best possible care for seniors experiencing age-related memory decline. In this subchapter, we will delve into the complexities of the aging brain and explore the various factors that contribute to memory changes in older adults.

Age-related memory decline is a natural part of the aging process. While it is normal to experience some forgetfulness as we get older, severe memory loss can be a sign of a more serious condition such as dementia or Alzheimer's disease. Understanding the differences between age-related memory decline, dementia, and Alzheimer's disease is crucial for caregivers to provide the appropriate support and care.

Mild cognitive impairment (MCI) is another common condition that affects seniors. It is characterized by a decline in cognitive abilities, including memory, that is noticeable but not severe enough to interfere with daily activities. Recognizing the signs of MCI and understanding its progression can help caregivers develop effective strategies to manage memory loss in seniors.

Prevention is always better than cure, and this holds true when it comes to memory loss in older adults. Implementing memory loss prevention strategies such as maintaining a healthy lifestyle, engaging in cognitive exercises, and managing chronic conditions can significantly reduce the risk of cognitive decline.

Memory training and cognitive exercises can be valuable tools in improving memory function in seniors. These exercises stimulate the brain and promote neuroplasticity, enhancing memory and cognitive abilities. Caregivers can incorporate memory training exercises into the daily routine of their seniors to help maintain and improve their memory function.

Medication and side effects can also play a role in memory loss in seniors. Certain medications, such as sedatives or anticholinergics, can affect memory and cognitive function. It is essential for caregivers to work closely with healthcare professionals to monitor medication usage and explore alternative options if necessary.

Nutritional deficiencies and sleep disorders can have a significant impact on memory function in older adults. Caregivers should ensure that their seniors have a well-balanced diet and address any sleep-related issues to promote optimal cognitive health.

Finally, coping strategies for caregivers are equally important in managing memory loss in seniors. Caregivers should foster a supportive and understanding environment, practice effective communication techniques, and seek support from community resources or support groups.

In conclusion, understanding the changes that occur in the aging brain and how they affect memory is crucial for caregivers. By implementing preventative strategies, engaging in memory training exercises, monitoring medication usage, addressing nutritional and sleep-related issues, and developing coping strategies, caregivers can provide the best possible care for seniors experiencing memory loss.

Differentiating Normal Memory Decline from Cognitive Impairment

As a caregiver for seniors with age-related memory decline, it is crucial to be able to differentiate between normal memory decline and cognitive impairment. Understanding the differences can help you provide the best care and support for your loved ones. In this subchapter, we will explore the various aspects of normal memory decline and cognitive impairment, providing you with valuable insights and practical tips.

Age-related memory decline is a natural part of the aging process. It is common for seniors to experience occasional forgetfulness, such as misplacing keys or forgetting appointments. Normal memory decline does not significantly impact daily functioning and does not interfere with independence. However, cognitive impairment, such as dementia or Alzheimer's disease, goes beyond normal forgetfulness.

Dementia is a progressive neurological disorder that affects memory, thinking, and behavior. It is characterized by a decline in cognitive abilities that impairs daily functioning. Alzheimer's disease, the most common form of dementia, causes memory loss, confusion, and changes in behavior. Mild cognitive impairment (MCI) is a stage between normal memory decline and dementia. Individuals with MCI may experience more significant memory problems than normal aging but do not meet the criteria for dementia.

To differentiate between normal memory decline and cognitive impairment, observe the following signs:

1. Frequency and severity: Normal memory decline is occasional and does not impact daily life significantly. Cognitive impairment involves frequent memory lapses and noticeable changes in behavior or personality.

2. Progression: Normal memory decline remains stable over time, while cognitive impairment worsens gradually.

3. Impact on daily activities: Normal memory decline does not interfere with daily tasks, while cognitive impairment hinders independence and requires assistance.

4. Recognition of familiar people and places: Individuals with normal memory decline recognize familiar faces and places. In cognitive impairment, there may be difficulty recognizing loved ones or familiar environments.

5. Language and communication skills: Normal memory decline does not affect language and communication abilities. In cognitive impairment, individuals may struggle to find words or follow conversations.

Understanding the differences between normal memory decline and cognitive impairment is essential for providing appropriate care. If you suspect cognitive impairment, it is crucial to seek medical evaluation and support. Early diagnosis can lead to effective management strategies and interventions.

In the next chapters, we will explore memory loss prevention strategies, memory training exercises, coping strategies for caregivers, and various factors that contribute to memory loss, such as medication side effects, nutritional deficiencies, and sleep disorders. By equipping yourself with knowledge and understanding, you can make a significant difference in the lives of seniors with age-related memory decline.

Common Causes of Age-Related Memory Decline

As caregivers, it is crucial to understand the common causes of age-related memory decline in order to provide the best care and support for seniors with memory impairments. This subchapter aims to shed light on the factors that contribute to memory decline in older adults and equip caregivers with the knowledge to address these issues effectively.

One of the primary causes of age-related memory decline is dementia, a condition characterized by a decline in cognitive abilities severe enough to interfere with daily life. Alzheimer's disease, the most common form of dementia, is especially prevalent among seniors. Caregivers need to be aware that memory loss is a hallmark symptom of Alzheimer's disease and should actively seek medical intervention for proper diagnosis and treatment.

Another condition that caregivers should be familiar with is mild cognitive impairment (MCI). Seniors with MCI experience a noticeable decline in memory and cognitive function, but it does not interfere significantly with their daily activities. It is crucial to monitor individuals with MCI closely, as they have a higher risk of developing dementia.

In addition to age-related conditions, certain medications and their side effects can also contribute to memory decline in older adults. Caregivers should be vigilant in monitoring any changes in memory or cognition after starting or altering medications, and consult with healthcare professionals if necessary.

Nutritional deficiencies can also play a role in memory decline. Poor diet and inadequate intake of essential nutrients can impair brain function, leading to memory problems. Caregivers should prioritize a balanced diet for their loved ones, including foods rich in omega-3 fatty acids, antioxidants, and B vitamins.

Sleep disorders, such as insomnia or sleep apnea, can have a detrimental effect on memory. Caregivers should ensure that seniors establish healthy sleep habits and create a conducive sleep environment to promote optimal cognitive function.

Lastly, this subchapter will explore coping strategies for caregivers to help seniors manage and adapt to memory loss. It will include practical tips such as creating routines, using memory aids and reminders, engaging in memory training exercises, and fostering social connections.

Understanding the common causes of age-related memory decline is crucial for caregivers to provide effective care and support to seniors with memory impairments. By addressing these causes and implementing appropriate strategies, caregivers can help improve the quality of life for their loved ones and promote overall cognitive health.

Chapter 2: Dementia and Memory Loss

Introduction to Dementia: Types and Symptoms

Dementia is a complex and progressive condition that affects millions of seniors worldwide. As caregivers, it is crucial for us to have a solid understanding of the different types of dementia and their associated symptoms. This knowledge will equip us to provide better care and support for our loved ones with age-related memory decline.

Dementia is not a single disease but rather a term that encompasses a range of conditions characterized by a decline in cognitive abilities. The most common type of dementia is Alzheimer's disease, accounting for approximately 60-80% of all cases. Other types include vascular dementia, Lewy body dementia, frontotemporal dementia, and mixed dementia, which is a combination of different types.

Each type of dementia is characterized by its unique set of symptoms. Alzheimer's disease typically presents with memory loss, confusion, difficulty with problem-solving, and changes in behavior and personality. Vascular dementia, on the other hand, is caused by reduced blood flow to the brain and often manifests as difficulty with planning, organizing, and making decisions.

Lewy body dementia is characterized by visual hallucinations, motor symptoms similar to Parkinson's disease, and fluctuations in cognitive abilities. Frontotemporal dementia primarily affects the frontal and temporal lobes of the brain, leading to changes in personality, language difficulties, and poor impulse control.

Recognizing the symptoms of dementia is crucial for early detection and intervention. Common symptoms include memory loss, difficulty with language and communication, confusion, impaired judgment, and changes in mood and behavior. However, it is important to remember that each individual may experience these symptoms differently, and the progression of dementia can vary widely.

As caregivers, it is essential to educate ourselves on the various types of dementia and their associated symptoms. This knowledge will help us understand the unique challenges our loved ones face and enable us to provide personalized care and support. Additionally, being aware of the different types of dementia can help us prepare for the future and seek appropriate medical and therapeutic interventions.

In the following chapters, we will delve deeper into each type of dementia, exploring its specific symptoms, progression, and potential treatment options. By gaining a comprehensive understanding of dementia, we can become better equipped to navigate the challenges of caregiving and provide the best possible care for our loved ones with age-related memory decline.

Understanding the Impact of Dementia on Memory

Dementia is a progressive neurological disorder that affects millions of seniors worldwide. As caregivers, it is crucial to comprehend the impact of dementia on memory in order to provide the best care and support for our loved ones. In this subchapter, we will explore the various ways in which dementia can affect memory and offer valuable insights on coping strategies for caregivers.

One of the most common forms of dementia is Alzheimer's disease, which is characterized by significant memory impairment. Individuals with Alzheimer's struggle to retain new information and often experience difficulties with short-term memory. They may forget conversations, appointments, or even the names of their loved ones. As caregivers, it is important to be patient and understanding, as repeated reminders and cues may be necessary to help them recall important details.

Another aspect of dementia's impact on memory is mild cognitive impairment. This condition is often a precursor to Alzheimer's disease and is marked by noticeable memory decline. Seniors with mild cognitive impairment may have difficulty with word retrieval, struggle to remember recent events, or misplace items frequently. Providing memory training exercises and cognitive stimulation can be beneficial in slowing down the progression of memory decline.

It is also important to be aware of the potential impact of medication and nutritional deficiencies on memory. Certain medications, such as sedatives or anticholinergics, can have side effects that affect cognitive function and memory. Nutritional deficiencies, particularly of vitamins B12 and D, can also contribute to memory loss in seniors. As caregivers, we must work closely with healthcare professionals to monitor medication usage and ensure that our loved ones have a balanced diet rich in essential nutrients.

Sleep disorders can also have a significant impact on memory in older adults. Conditions like insomnia or sleep apnea can disrupt the quality of sleep and impair memory consolidation. Establishing a regular sleep routine and creating a conducive sleep environment can help seniors improve their sleep patterns and consequently enhance their memory function.

Lastly, in this subchapter, we will discuss coping strategies for caregivers dealing with the challenges of memory loss in seniors. We will explore techniques such as creating memory aids, using visual cues, and implementing daily routines to provide structure and support. Additionally, we will delve into the importance of self-care for caregivers, as navigating the complexities of dementia care can be emotionally and physically demanding.

Understanding the impact of dementia on memory is essential for caregivers. By gaining insights into the various aspects of memory decline in seniors, we can provide the necessary support, implement preventive strategies, and enhance the overall well-being of our loved ones.

Managing Memory Loss in Individuals with Dementia

Memory loss is a common and distressing symptom among individuals with dementia. As a caregiver, it is crucial to understand how to effectively manage memory loss in order to provide the best possible care for your loved one. This subchapter will explore various strategies and techniques that caregivers can employ to support individuals with dementia in coping with their memory decline.

One important aspect of managing memory loss in individuals with dementia is creating a structured and organized environment. By establishing routines and maintaining a consistent schedule, you can help your loved one feel more secure and reduce their anxiety. Labeling items and using memory aids, such as calendars and to-do lists, can also assist in compensating for memory deficits.

Memory training and cognitive exercises can be beneficial for individuals with dementia. Engaging in activities that stimulate the brain, such as puzzles, word games, and memory exercises, can help maintain cognitive function and slow down the progression of memory decline. Additionally, incorporating physical exercise into their daily routine has been shown to improve memory and overall brain health.

It is important to be aware of the potential side effects of medications that may contribute to memory loss. Consult with your loved one's healthcare provider to evaluate the medication regimen and discuss any concerns regarding memory impairment. In some cases, alternative medications or dosage adjustments may be considered to minimize memory-related side effects.

Nutritional deficiencies and sleep disorders can also impact memory in seniors. Ensuring a well-balanced diet that includes brain-healthy foods, such as fruits, vegetables, whole grains, and omega-3 fatty acids, can support optimal brain function.

Additionally, addressing any sleep disturbances, such as insomnia or sleep apnea, can improve memory and cognitive abilities.

Coping with memory loss can be challenging for both individuals with dementia and their caregivers. It is important to practice patience, empathy, and understanding. Encourage open communication and provide emotional support to your loved one. Seek out support groups or professional counseling services to help you navigate the emotional aspects of caregiving.

In conclusion, managing memory loss in individuals with dementia requires a comprehensive approach that encompasses environmental modifications, cognitive exercises, medication evaluation, nutritional support, and emotional care. By implementing these strategies, caregivers can enhance their loved one's quality of life and create a supportive and nurturing environment for those with age-related memory decline.

Chapter 3: Alzheimer's Disease and Memory Impairment

Overview of Alzheimer's Disease: Causes and Progression

Title: Overview of Alzheimer's Disease: Causes and Progression

Introduction:

In this subchapter, we will provide an in-depth understanding of Alzheimer's disease, its causes, and how it progresses over time. As caregivers of seniors with age-related memory decline, it is crucial to have a comprehensive knowledge of Alzheimer's disease, as it is one of the most prevalent causes of memory impairment and dementia. By understanding its causes and progression, caregivers can better support their loved ones and develop effective strategies to manage the challenges associated with this condition.

Causes of Alzheimer's Disease:

Alzheimer's disease is a complex neurological disorder that is primarily characterized by the accumulation of abnormal protein deposits in the brain, leading to the death of brain cells. While the exact cause remains unknown, several factors contribute to its development, such as age, genetics, lifestyle choices, and environmental factors. Caregivers should be aware of these potential causes to help identify the risk factors and take preventive measures when possible.

Progression of Alzheimer's Disease:

Alzheimer's disease typically progresses in stages, each with distinct symptoms and challenges. The early stage is often characterized by mild memory loss and difficulty in finding words or organizing thoughts. As the disease advances, individuals may experience increased confusion, personality changes, and difficulties with daily tasks. In the later stages, individuals may require round-the-clock care, as they lose the ability to communicate, recognize loved ones, and perform basic self-care activities. Understanding the progression of Alzheimer's disease is essential for caregivers to anticipate and address the changing needs of their loved ones.

Impact on Seniors and Caregivers:

Alzheimer's disease not only affects seniors but also has a significant impact on their caregivers. Caregivers may experience emotional and physical exhaustion, stress, and feelings of helplessness as they witness the decline of their loved ones. It is crucial for caregivers to prioritize self-care and seek support to navigate the challenges associated with caring for someone with Alzheimer's disease.

Conclusion:

This subchapter has provided an overview of Alzheimer's disease, its causes, and progression. As caregivers, it is vital to educate ourselves about this disease to better support our loved ones who are experiencing age-related memory decline. By understanding the causes and progression of Alzheimer's disease, caregivers can develop effective coping strategies, seek appropriate medical interventions, and enhance the quality of life for both seniors and themselves.

Memory Impairment in Alzheimer's Disease

Alzheimer's disease is a progressive brain disorder that affects millions of seniors worldwide. As a caregiver, it is crucial to understand the impact this disease has on memory and how to support your loved one throughout their journey. This subchapter delves into the topic of memory impairment in Alzheimer's disease, providing you with valuable insights and strategies to navigate this challenging aspect of caregiving.

Memory loss is one of the earliest and most prominent symptoms of Alzheimer's disease. As the disease progresses, individuals may experience difficulty remembering recent events, conversations, or even the names of their loved ones. This can be distressing for both the person with Alzheimer's and their caregiver. Understanding the underlying mechanisms of memory impairment in Alzheimer's is essential to providing effective care.

In Alzheimer's disease, memory impairment primarily affects the hippocampus, a region of the brain responsible for forming and retrieving memories. As the disease progresses, other areas of the brain involved in memory, such as the frontal cortex, are also affected. This leads to further decline in memory function and other cognitive abilities.

While it may be disheartening to witness your loved one's memory decline, there are strategies you can employ to support them. Memory training and cognitive exercises can help slow down the progression of memory impairment and improve overall cognitive function. Encouraging your loved one to engage in activities that stimulate their memory, such as puzzles, word games, or reminiscing about past events, can be beneficial.

Additionally, it is important to pay attention to lifestyle factors that may contribute to memory impairment. Poor sleep quality, medication side effects, and nutritional deficiencies can all impact memory function. Ensuring your loved one maintains a healthy sleep pattern, reviewing their medications with their healthcare provider, and providing a well-balanced diet rich in essential nutrients can help mitigate memory loss.

As a caregiver, coping with memory impairment in Alzheimer's disease can be challenging. It is crucial to adopt coping strategies that prioritize your own well-being while supporting your loved one. Seeking support from other caregivers, joining support groups, and practicing self-care are essential components of navigating this journey.

In conclusion, memory impairment is a significant aspect of Alzheimer's disease that caregivers must understand and address. By employing memory training techniques, managing lifestyle factors, and implementing coping strategies, you can provide the best possible care for your loved one with Alzheimer's disease.

Strategies for Supporting Memory in Individuals with Alzheimer's

Introduction:

Memory loss is a common symptom of Alzheimer's disease and can be challenging for both individuals with the condition and their caregivers. However, there are strategies and techniques that caregivers can employ to support memory and enhance the quality of life for their loved ones. This subchapter explores various approaches to help individuals with Alzheimer's maintain their cognitive abilities and improve their overall well-being.

1. Establish a Routine:

Creating a daily routine can provide structure and familiarity, which can be beneficial for individuals with Alzheimer's. Ensure that activities such as meals, medication administration, and exercise occur at the same time each day. This routine can help individuals feel more secure and minimize confusion.

2. Use Memory Aids:

Memory aids, such as calendars, medication organizers, and reminder apps, can help individuals with Alzheimer's remember important dates, appointments, and tasks. Encourage the use of these aids and regularly check and update them together.

3. Simplify the Environment:

Minimize distractions by keeping the environment clutter-free and well-organized. Labeling drawers, cupboards, and other frequently used items can help individuals locate objects independently. Use contrasting colors for visual cues and ensure adequate lighting to enhance visibility.

4. Encourage Exercise and Mental Stimulation:

Physical exercise has shown to have positive effects on cognition and memory. Encourage regular exercise tailored to the individual's abilities, such as walking or gentle stretching. Engage in mentally stimulating activities such as puzzles, reading, or engaging in hobbies to keep the mind active.

5. Maintain a Nutritious Diet:

Certain nutrients, such as omega-3 fatty acids and antioxidants, have been linked to brain health. Ensure that the individual consumes a balanced diet rich in fruits, vegetables, whole grains, and lean proteins. Consult with a healthcare professional or a registered dietitian for personalized dietary recommendations.

6. Foster Social Connections:

Social interactions can help stimulate memory and prevent feelings of isolation. Encourage individuals to participate in group activities, join support groups, or engage in community programs tailored for individuals with Alzheimer's. Regular visits from family and friends can also provide emotional support.

7. Practice Patience and Empathy:

Dealing with memory loss can be frustrating for both individuals with Alzheimer's and their caregivers. Practice patience, empathy, and understanding. Use clear and simple language, provide visual cues, and allow extra time for tasks. Celebrate small successes and focus on maintaining a positive and supportive environment.

Conclusion:

Supporting memory in individuals with Alzheimer's requires a multifaceted approach that includes establishing routines, utilizing memory aids, simplifying the environment, encouraging exercise and mental stimulation, maintaining a nutritious diet, fostering social connections, and practicing patience and empathy. By implementing these strategies, caregivers can help individuals with Alzheimer's maintain their cognitive abilities and improve their overall quality of life.

Chapter 4: Mild Cognitive Impairment in Seniors

Recognizing Mild Cognitive Impairment: Signs and Symptoms

As a caregiver, it is crucial to understand the signs and symptoms of mild cognitive impairment (MCI) in seniors with age-related memory decline. Recognizing these early warning signs can help you provide the necessary support and care for your loved one. In this subchapter, we will explore the various signs and symptoms of MCI and how they differ from normal age-related memory decline.

MCI is often considered a transitional stage between normal cognitive aging and dementia. While individuals with MCI may experience memory problems, they generally remain independent in their daily activities. However, it is important to note that MCI can progress to dementia if not addressed properly.

One of the primary signs of MCI is memory loss that is more noticeable than typical age-related forgetfulness. Seniors with MCI may frequently forget important events or conversations, struggle to remember recently learned information, or rely heavily on notes and reminders. They may also have difficulty concentrating and may take longer to complete tasks.

Another common symptom of MCI is language difficulties. Seniors may have trouble finding the right words during conversations or struggle with expressing their thoughts coherently. They may also experience difficulties with spatial awareness, such as getting lost in familiar places or having difficulty navigating.

Changes in mood and personality are also common in individuals with MCI. They may become more irritable, anxious, or withdrawn. Depression is also more prevalent in seniors with MCI, as they may struggle with the changes in their cognitive abilities.

It is important to keep in mind that everyone's experience with MCI can vary, and not all individuals will exhibit the same symptoms. However, if you notice any significant changes in your loved one's cognitive abilities or behavior, it is essential to consult with a healthcare professional for a proper evaluation and diagnosis.

In the next subchapter, we will discuss memory loss prevention strategies for older adults and memory training exercises that can help maintain cognitive function. By understanding the signs and symptoms of MCI, you can take proactive steps to provide the necessary support and care for your loved one, ultimately improving their quality of life.

Memory Challenges Associated with Mild Cognitive Impairment

Mild Cognitive Impairment (MCI) is a condition that affects many seniors and is often considered a transitional stage between normal aging and dementia. As caregivers, it is important to understand the memory challenges associated with MCI and how to support our loved ones through this phase. In this subchapter, we will explore the specific memory difficulties seniors with MCI may face and provide strategies to help caregivers navigate these challenges.

One common memory challenge associated with MCI is forgetfulness. Seniors with MCI may experience difficulty remembering recent conversations, appointments, or events. They may also have trouble recalling names or faces of people they have just met. As caregivers, it is essential to be patient and understanding when our loved ones struggle with forgetfulness. We can assist by providing reminders, using calendars or sticky notes, and establishing routines to help them stay organized.

Another memory challenge seniors with MCI may encounter is difficulty with prospective memory. Prospective memory refers to remembering to do things in the future, such as taking medication or attending appointments. Caregivers can support seniors with MCI by using reminders, setting up pill organizers, and helping them establish a daily routine to ensure important tasks are not forgotten.

Furthermore, seniors with MCI may struggle with word-finding difficulties, also known as tip-of-the-tongue phenomenon. They may have difficulty recalling words or finding the right words to express themselves. As caregivers, we can offer gentle prompts or suggestions to help them find the words they are searching for. Patience and active listening are key when supporting our loved ones through this challenge.

It is important to note that memory challenges associated with MCI vary from person to person. Some individuals may experience more severe memory impairments, while others may have relatively mild difficulties. As caregivers, our role is to provide support and understanding tailored to our loved one's specific needs.

By recognizing and understanding the memory challenges associated with MCI, caregivers can implement effective strategies to assist their loved ones. These strategies include providing reminders, establishing routines, using calendars and pill organizers, offering gentle prompts for word-finding difficulties, and practicing patience and active listening.

In the next subchapter, we will explore memory loss prevention strategies for older adults and memory training exercises that can benefit seniors with MCI. Stay tuned for valuable information and practical tips to help enhance and preserve memory function in our aging loved ones.

Cognitive Interventions for Managing Mild Cognitive Impairment

Mild cognitive impairment (MCI) is a condition that affects many seniors and can be challenging for both the individuals experiencing it and their caregivers. However, there are various cognitive interventions that can help manage and even slow down the progression of MCI. In this subchapter, we will explore some effective strategies and techniques that caregivers can implement to support their loved ones with MCI.

One of the most important cognitive interventions for managing MCI is memory training and cognitive exercises. These exercises can help improve memory, attention, and problem-solving skills. Encourage your loved one to engage in activities such as puzzles, memory games, and brain-training apps. These exercises not only stimulate the brain but also provide a sense of accomplishment and boost self-confidence.

In addition to cognitive exercises, it is crucial to address any underlying medical conditions that may contribute to memory decline. Certain medications and nutritional deficiencies can affect cognitive function. Therefore, it is essential to consult with a healthcare professional to review your loved one's medication regimen and ensure they are receiving proper nutrition. By addressing these factors, you can potentially alleviate or even reverse some of the cognitive impairment.

Another area that caregivers should focus on is promoting good sleep hygiene. Sleep disorders, such as insomnia or sleep apnea, can significantly impact memory and cognitive function. Encourage your loved one to establish a regular sleep schedule, create a comfortable sleep environment, and practice relaxation techniques before bed. Adequate sleep can enhance memory consolidation and overall cognitive performance.

Coping strategies are also essential for both the individuals with MCI and their caregivers. Encourage your loved one to use memory aids, such as calendars, reminder apps, and notes, to compensate for any memory deficits. Help them establish a daily routine and provide structure to their day. Breaking tasks into smaller, manageable steps can also make it easier for them to complete daily activities.

Lastly, as a caregiver, it is important to take care of yourself as well. Caring for someone with MCI can be emotionally and physically demanding. Seek support from support groups or therapy to help manage stress and burnout. Remember to prioritize self-care and take breaks when needed.

In conclusion, cognitive interventions play a vital role in managing mild cognitive impairment. By incorporating memory training and cognitive exercises, addressing underlying medical conditions, promoting good sleep hygiene, and implementing coping strategies, caregivers can provide effective support to their loved ones. Remember that managing MCI is a journey, and with patience, understanding, and the right interventions, individuals with MCI can lead fulfilling lives.

Chapter 5: Memory Loss Prevention Strategies for Older Adults

Maintaining Brain Health: Lifestyle Factors and Memory

In this subchapter, we will explore the crucial role that lifestyle factors play in maintaining brain health and memory in seniors with age-related memory decline. As caregivers, it is essential for us to understand how we can support our loved ones in adopting healthy habits that can positively impact their cognitive function. By implementing these strategies, we can help delay or even prevent further memory decline.

1. Physical Exercise: Regular physical activity has been shown to improve brain health and memory. Encourage your loved ones to engage in activities such as walking, swimming, or yoga. These exercises not only enhance blood flow to the brain but also stimulate the growth of new neurons.

2. Mental Stimulation: Engaging in mentally stimulating activities is like exercise for the brain. Encourage your loved ones to read books, solve puzzles, play chess, or engage in other activities that require cognitive effort. This can help strengthen neural connections and improve memory.

3. Healthy Diet: A well-balanced diet plays a significant role in brain health. Encourage your loved ones to consume foods rich in antioxidants, omega-3 fatty acids, and vitamins such as B12 and D. These nutrients have been linked to improved cognitive function and memory.

4. Quality Sleep: Sufficient sleep is vital for memory consolidation. Help your loved ones establish a regular sleep routine by creating a peaceful environment, limiting caffeine intake, and encouraging relaxation techniques before bedtime.

5. Social Engagement: Social interaction is not only beneficial for emotional well-being but also for brain health. Encourage your loved ones to maintain relationships, participate in group activities, or volunteer. These interactions stimulate the brain and help preserve memory function.

6. Medication and Side Effects: Be aware of the potential memory side effects of certain medications. Consult with healthcare professionals to discuss alternative medications or dosage adjustments that may minimize memory decline.

7. Nutritional Deficiencies: Address any nutritional deficiencies that may contribute to memory loss. Encourage your loved ones to consume a varied diet rich in fruits, vegetables, whole grains, and lean proteins. Consider consulting with a dietician to ensure proper nutrient intake.

8. Coping Strategies: Help your loved ones develop coping strategies to manage memory loss. Encourage the use of memory aids such as calendars, reminder apps, and medication organizers. These tools can help compensate for memory deficits and maintain independence.

By focusing on these lifestyle factors, caregivers can make a significant difference in the brain health and memory of seniors with age-related memory decline. Implementing these strategies will not only support cognitive function but also enhance the overall well-being of our loved ones. Remember, every small step towards maintaining brain health matters and can lead to a better quality of life for those we care for.

Engaging in Physical and Mental Activities to Preserve Memory

As a caregiver for seniors with age-related memory decline, you play a crucial role in helping your loved ones maintain their cognitive abilities and preserve their memory. One of the most effective ways to achieve this is by encouraging them to engage in physical and mental activities regularly. In this subchapter, we will explore the various strategies and techniques that can be used to promote memory preservation through these activities.

Physical exercise has been proven to have numerous benefits for the brain and overall cognitive function. Encourage your loved ones to engage in activities such as walking, swimming, dancing, or even gardening. These exercises help increase blood flow to the brain, stimulate the growth of new neurons, and improve memory and cognitive function. Additionally, regular physical activity can also reduce the risk of developing conditions such as dementia and Alzheimer's disease.

In addition to physical exercise, mental activities are equally important in preserving memory. Engaging in activities that challenge the mind can help maintain cognitive abilities and improve memory. Encourage your loved ones to participate in brain-stimulating activities such as puzzles, crosswords, reading, learning a new skill or language, or playing memory-enhancing games. These activities keep the brain active, improve concentration, and enhance memory function.

Memory training and cognitive exercises specifically designed for seniors can also be beneficial. These exercises focus on memory retention and retrieval techniques, helping seniors improve their memory and cognitive abilities. Encourage your loved ones to participate in memory training programs, either in a group setting or through online platforms that offer interactive exercises and games.

It is important to be aware that certain medications and nutritional deficiencies can impact memory in seniors. If your loved one is experiencing memory loss as a side effect of medication or due to nutritional deficiencies, consult their healthcare provider to explore alternative options or supplements that can help mitigate these effects.

Lastly, prioritize a good night's sleep for your loved ones. Sleep disorders can contribute to memory problems and cognitive decline. Establish a consistent sleep routine, create a comfortable sleep environment, and encourage relaxation techniques such as meditation or gentle exercise before bedtime.

By encouraging your loved ones to engage in physical and mental activities, you are actively helping them preserve their memory and cognitive function. Remember to be patient and supportive throughout the process, and celebrate even small improvements. Your dedication as a caregiver is invaluable in ensuring your loved one's overall well-being and quality of life.

Adopting a Healthy Diet for Cognitive Function

As caregivers of seniors with age-related memory decline, it is crucial for us to understand the impact of diet on cognitive function. The food we consume plays a significant role in maintaining brain health and can greatly influence memory and overall cognitive abilities. In this subchapter, we will explore the importance of adopting a healthy diet for cognitive function and provide practical tips for implementing dietary changes.

Age-related memory decline, dementia, Alzheimer's disease, and mild cognitive impairment are conditions that can greatly affect a senior's quality of life. While there is no cure for these conditions, research suggests that a healthy diet can help slow down cognitive decline and improve memory.

First and foremost, it is essential to focus on a balanced diet that includes a variety of fruits, vegetables, whole grains, lean proteins, and healthy fats. These foods provide essential nutrients such as antioxidants, vitamins, and omega-3 fatty acids that promote brain health. Encourage your loved one to consume colorful fruits and vegetables, such as berries, leafy greens, and cruciferous vegetables, as they are rich in antioxidants and have been associated with improved cognitive function.

Another aspect to consider is reducing the intake of processed foods, sugary snacks, and saturated fats. These foods are linked to inflammation and oxidative stress, which can negatively impact cognitive function. Instead, opt for healthier alternatives, such as nuts, seeds, olive oil, and fish, which are high in omega-3 fatty acids and have been shown to support brain health.

Furthermore, ensure that your loved one stays hydrated throughout the day. Dehydration can lead to cognitive impairments, so encourage them to drink plenty of water and limit the intake of caffeinated beverages.

Supplements can also play a role in maintaining cognitive function, but it is important to consult a healthcare professional before incorporating them into your loved one's routine. Omega-3 fatty acid supplements, B vitamins, and antioxidants like vitamin E and C have shown potential benefits for brain health.

Lastly, remember that adopting a healthy diet is not just about the food itself but also about creating a positive eating environment. Encourage regular mealtimes, engage in meaningful conversations during meals, and make the dining experience enjoyable for your loved one.

By adopting a healthy diet for cognitive function, caregivers can play a vital role in supporting their loved ones' brain health. While dietary changes alone may not reverse memory decline, they can contribute to overall well-being and potentially slow down cognitive decline. Remember to consult with a healthcare professional or nutritionist to tailor the diet to individual needs and preferences.

Chapter 6: Memory Training and Cognitive Exercises for Seniors

Importance of Cognitive Stimulation for Memory Enhancement

Introduction:

As caregivers of seniors with age-related memory decline, it is crucial for us to understand the importance of cognitive stimulation in enhancing memory. Memory loss can be challenging for both the individuals experiencing it and their caregivers. However, by incorporating memory training and cognitive exercises into their daily routine, we can help seniors maintain and improve their memory function. This subchapter will explore the significance of cognitive stimulation and provide practical strategies for enhancing memory in older adults.

Benefits of Cognitive Stimulation:

1. Delaying Cognitive Decline: Engaging in cognitive activities stimulates the brain and can slow down the progression of age-related memory decline. Regular mental exercises help in building cognitive reserve, which acts as a buffer against cognitive impairment.

2. Improving Memory Function: Cognitive stimulation exercises focus on memory enhancement, attention, and problem-solving skills. By challenging the brain through activities such as puzzles, memory games, or reading, seniors can improve their ability to retain and recall information.

3. Enhancing Quality of Life: Maintaining cognitive abilities allows seniors to maintain their independence and actively participate in daily activities. It boosts their self-esteem, confidence, and overall well-being.

Strategies for Cognitive Stimulation:

1. Memory Training: Encourage seniors to engage in memory training exercises specifically designed to target memory enhancement. These can include repeating information, visualization techniques, and using mnemonic devices.

2. Cognitive Exercises: Engaging in activities that require mental effort, such as crossword puzzles, Sudoku, or learning a new skill, can help seniors exercise their cognitive abilities. Encourage them to participate in these activities regularly.

3. Social Interaction: Social engagement promotes cognitive stimulation. Encourage seniors to participate in group activities, join clubs or organizations, or spend time with family and friends. These interactions stimulate memory recall and provide opportunities for mental stimulation.

4. Physical Exercise: Regular physical exercise has been linked to improved cognitive function. Encourage seniors to engage in activities such as walking, dancing, or yoga, as they can enhance blood flow to the brain and support memory enhancement.

Conclusion:

Cognitive stimulation plays a vital role in memory enhancement for older adults with age-related memory decline. As caregivers, it is essential to incorporate memory training exercises, cognitive activities, social interaction, and physical exercise into their daily routine. By doing so, we can help seniors maintain their cognitive abilities, slow down cognitive decline, and improve their overall quality of life. Remember, every effort counts when it comes to supporting our loved ones in their memory journey.

Memory Training Techniques and Programs

Memory decline is a common concern for caregivers of seniors, especially those who are dealing with age-related memory decline, dementia, Alzheimer's disease, or mild cognitive impairment. As a caregiver, it is essential to understand the various memory training techniques and programs available to help seniors maintain and improve their cognitive abilities. This subchapter will explore different strategies and programs aimed at preventing memory loss, improving memory function, and coping with memory impairment in older adults.

One effective memory training technique is cognitive exercises. These exercises are designed to challenge and stimulate the brain, improving memory and cognitive function. Examples of cognitive exercises include puzzles, word games, memory games, and brain training apps. These exercises can be easily incorporated into a senior's daily routine and can be tailored to their individual needs and abilities.

Memory training programs are another valuable resource for caregivers. These programs are specifically designed to target memory impairment and provide structured training to improve memory function. Programs such as the Memory Improvement Program and the Memory Fitness Program offer comprehensive training modules that focus on memory techniques, strategies, and exercises. These programs can be conducted in a group setting or individually, depending on the senior's preferences and needs.

In addition to cognitive exercises and training programs, caregivers should also be aware of the impact of medication, nutritional deficiencies, and sleep disorders on memory function. Certain medications can cause memory loss as a side effect, and nutritional deficiencies can impair cognitive abilities. Sleep disorders, such as insomnia or sleep apnea, can also contribute to memory problems. It is crucial for caregivers to work closely with healthcare professionals to address these underlying issues and develop a holistic approach to memory care.

Finally, coping strategies for caregivers are essential in managing the challenges associated with memory loss in seniors. These strategies may include creating a memory-friendly environment, using memory aids such as calendars and reminder systems, practicing effective communication techniques, and seeking support from support groups or counseling services. By implementing these coping strategies, caregivers can reduce stress and better support their loved ones with memory impairment.

In conclusion, memory training techniques and programs play a vital role in supporting seniors with age-related memory decline, dementia, or Alzheimer's disease. By incorporating cognitive exercises, participating in memory training programs, addressing underlying issues, and implementing effective coping strategies, caregivers can help seniors maintain and improve their memory function. Understanding and utilizing these techniques and programs can significantly enhance the quality of life for both seniors and their caregivers.

Incorporating Cognitive Exercises into Daily Routines

As a caregiver for a senior with age-related memory decline, you play a crucial role in supporting their cognitive health and overall well-being. One effective way to do this is by incorporating cognitive exercises into their daily routines. By engaging in these activities regularly, you can help stimulate their brain, improve memory functions, and slow down the progression of memory decline.

There are numerous cognitive exercises that you can incorporate into your loved one's daily routine. These exercises target various cognitive domains such as attention, memory, problem-solving, and language skills. Here are a few examples:

1. Puzzle Time: Encourage your loved one to solve puzzles like crosswords, Sudoku, or jigsaw puzzles. These activities challenge their problem-solving skills and improve concentration and memory.

2. Memory Games: Play memory games with your loved one, such as matching cards or recalling a list of items. This helps enhance their short-term memory and concentration abilities.

3. Reading and Discussion: Set aside time each day for reading. Encourage your loved one to read books, newspapers, or

magazines, and engage in discussions about the content. This helps improve their comprehension and language skills.

4. Brain Training Apps: Explore the various brain training apps available that offer a range of cognitive exercises. These apps are designed to challenge different cognitive functions and can be a fun and interactive way for your loved one to exercise their brain.

5. Learning a New Skill: Encourage your loved one to learn something new, such as playing a musical instrument, painting, or gardening. Learning a new skill engages multiple areas of the brain and can improve memory and cognitive abilities.

It's important to remember that incorporating cognitive exercises should be done gradually and tailored to your loved one's abilities and interests. Start with simple exercises and gradually increase the complexity as they progress. Be patient and provide encouragement and support throughout the process.

Incorporating cognitive exercises into daily routines is just one piece of the puzzle in caring for a senior with memory decline. It's essential to combine these exercises with other memory loss prevention strategies such as a healthy diet, regular exercise, sufficient sleep, and social engagement. By adopting a holistic approach, you can provide the best possible care and support for your loved one's cognitive health.

Chapter 7: Memory Loss Due to Medication and Side Effects

Medications That Can Impair Memory Function

As caregivers of seniors with age-related memory decline, it is crucial for you to be aware of the potential impact medications can have on memory function. Many commonly prescribed drugs can interfere with cognitive abilities, leading to memory loss and other forms of cognitive decline. In this subchapter, we will delve into the medications that can impair memory function, providing you with the knowledge to better navigate your loved one's medication regimen.

One of the most well-known classes of medications that can affect memory function is benzodiazepines. These drugs, often prescribed for anxiety and sleep disorders, work by depressing the central nervous system. While they can provide short-term relief, their long-term use has been linked to memory impairment in seniors. It is important to work closely with your loved one's healthcare provider to monitor the dosage and duration of benzodiazepine use.

Another category of medications that may impact memory function is anticholinergic drugs. These include certain antihistamines, antidepressants, and medications for overactive bladder. Anticholinergics work by blocking the action of acetylcholine, a neurotransmitter involved in learning and memory. While these medications can be necessary for specific conditions, prolonged use may contribute to memory problems.

Consult with your loved one's doctor to explore alternative options or to adjust dosages if necessary.

It is also essential to be aware of the potential memory-related side effects of other commonly prescribed drugs, such as statins (used to manage cholesterol), certain blood pressure medications, and anti-seizure drugs. While these medications are often vital for managing various health conditions, they may have unintended consequences on memory function. Regular communication with the healthcare team is crucial to assess the benefits and risks of these medications for your loved one.

In addition to understanding the medications that can impair memory function, it is equally important to explore strategies for memory loss prevention. Encouraging a healthy lifestyle, including regular exercise, a balanced diet, and adequate sleep, can support cognitive health. Engaging older adults in memory training and cognitive exercises can also help maintain and improve memory function.

As caregivers, it is essential to stay informed about the medications your loved one is taking and their potential effects on memory. Open communication with healthcare providers, regular medication reviews, and exploring alternative options when possible can all play a role in minimizing the impact of medication on memory function.

By arming yourself with knowledge and working closely with healthcare professionals, you can better support your loved one in managing age-related memory decline while minimizing the potential negative impact of medications. Remember, you are not alone in this journey, and there are resources available to help you navigate the complexities of caregiving for seniors with memory decline.

Understanding the Side Effects of Common Medications

Medications play a crucial role in managing the various health conditions that seniors may face, including age-related memory decline, dementia, Alzheimer's disease, and mild cognitive impairment. However, it is important for caregivers to be aware of the potential side effects that these medications may cause, as they can sometimes have an impact on memory and cognitive function.

One common side effect of certain medications is memory loss. Some drugs used to treat anxiety, depression, and sleep disorders, known as benzodiazepines, can impair memory and cognitive function in older adults. These medications may cause confusion, drowsiness, and difficulty concentrating, which can all contribute to memory problems. It is important for caregivers to monitor the effects of these medications and discuss any concerns with the prescribing doctor.

In addition to benzodiazepines, anticholinergic medications are another class of drugs that can affect memory. These drugs are commonly used to treat conditions such as allergies, motion sickness, and urinary incontinence. However, they can also cause confusion, memory loss, and cognitive decline in seniors. Caregivers should be cautious when seniors are prescribed anticholinergic medications and discuss alternative options with the doctor if memory problems arise.

Furthermore, certain medications used to manage chronic conditions like high blood pressure, diabetes, and cholesterol can also have an impact on memory. Some of these drugs, such as statins, have been associated with memory loss and cognitive decline in some individuals. It is crucial for caregivers to be aware of these potential side effects and communicate with the healthcare provider if they suspect any memory problems related to these medications.

In addition to medication side effects, nutritional deficiencies and sleep disorders can also contribute to memory loss in older adults. Caregivers should ensure that seniors are getting a well-balanced diet and taking any necessary nutritional supplements. Adequate sleep is also vital for memory consolidation, so caregivers should address any sleep disturbances or disorders that seniors may be experiencing.

In conclusion, understanding the potential side effects of common medications is essential for caregivers of seniors with age-related memory decline. Medications such as benzodiazepines and anticholinergic drugs can impair memory and cognitive function. Additionally, certain medications used to manage chronic conditions may also have an impact on memory. Nutritional deficiencies and sleep disorders can further contribute to memory loss. Caregivers should closely monitor the effects of medications, address any nutritional deficiencies, and ensure seniors are getting adequate sleep to support their memory and cognitive health.

Strategies for Minimizing Medication-Related Memory Loss

As a caregiver for seniors with age-related memory decline, it is crucial to understand the potential impact of medication on memory function. Medication-related memory loss is a common concern among older adults, especially those with dementia, Alzheimer's disease, or mild cognitive impairment. This subchapter will provide you with practical strategies to help minimize medication-related memory loss and improve the overall well-being of your loved one.

1. Communication with healthcare professionals: Open and clear communication with your loved one's healthcare team is essential. Make sure to inform them about any memory issues or concerns related to medication. They can review the prescribed medications and assess if any alternative options or dosage adjustments are possible to minimize memory-related side effects.

2. Regular medication reviews: Schedule regular medication reviews with your loved one's healthcare provider. This will help ensure that the medications being taken are necessary and appropriate. Sometimes, medications can be discontinued or replaced with alternatives that have fewer cognitive side effects.

3. Consistent medication routine: Create a consistent medication routine to help your loved one remember to take their medications. Use pill organizers or smartphone reminder apps to help them stay on track. Avoid making changes to their medication schedule without consulting their healthcare provider.

4. Lifestyle modifications: Encourage your loved one to adopt a healthy lifestyle that supports memory function. This includes regular exercise, a balanced diet rich in fruits and vegetables, adequate sleep, and stress management techniques. These lifestyle modifications can have a positive impact on memory and overall cognitive health.

5. Memory training and cognitive exercises: Engage your loved one in memory training and cognitive exercises. These activities can help improve memory and cognitive function. Encourage them to engage in puzzles, memory games, reading, and social activities that stimulate their brain.

6. Nutritional supplements: Discuss with the healthcare provider the possibility of incorporating nutritional supplements that support memory and cognitive health. Omega-3 fatty acids, vitamin B12, and antioxidants are among the supplements that have shown potential benefits in improving memory function.

7. Regular sleep schedule: Ensure that your loved one maintains a regular sleep schedule. Poor sleep quality can significantly impact memory function. Encourage a relaxing bedtime routine and a comfortable sleep environment.

Remember, every individual is unique, and what works for one person may not work for another. It is essential to monitor the effects of any strategies implemented and make adjustments as necessary. By being proactive and implementing these strategies, you can help minimize medication-related memory loss and improve the overall quality of life for your loved one with age-related memory decline.

Chapter 8: Memory Loss and Nutritional Deficiencies in Seniors

Nutrition and Memory: Essential Nutrients for Brain Health

As a caregiver for seniors with age-related memory decline, it is essential to understand the relationship between nutrition and memory. The food we consume plays a significant role in maintaining brain health and can have a direct impact on memory function. In this subchapter, we will explore the essential nutrients that support brain health and memory in older adults.

One key nutrient for brain health is omega-3 fatty acids. These healthy fats are abundant in certain types of fish, such as salmon, mackerel, and sardines. Omega-3 fatty acids have been shown to reduce inflammation in the brain and promote the growth of new brain cells, which can enhance memory and cognitive function.

Another important nutrient is antioxidants, which help protect the brain from oxidative stress and damage caused by free radicals. Colorful fruits and vegetables, such as berries, spinach, and kale, are rich in antioxidants and should be included in the senior's diet. Additionally, consuming foods high in vitamin E, such as nuts and seeds, can also contribute to brain health.

B vitamins, particularly vitamin B12 and folate, are essential for maintaining healthy brain function. Deficiencies in these vitamins can lead to memory problems and cognitive decline. Good sources of vitamin B12 include meat, fish, eggs, and dairy products, while folate can be found in leafy greens, legumes, and fortified grains.

Incorporating a balanced diet that includes these essential nutrients can help prevent memory loss and support overall brain health in seniors. However, it is important to note that nutritional deficiencies can still occur even with a healthy diet. Certain medications, such as those used to manage chronic conditions, can interfere with nutrient absorption. Therefore, it is crucial to consult with a healthcare professional to address any potential nutritional deficiencies and explore supplementation if necessary.

As a caregiver, you can also promote good sleep hygiene, as sleep disorders can contribute to memory problems. Encourage a regular sleep schedule and create a calming bedtime routine to help seniors get a restful night's sleep.

Remember, nutrition is a crucial aspect of maintaining brain health and preventing memory decline in older adults. By understanding the essential nutrients and incorporating them into the senior's diet, you can play an active role in supporting their cognitive well-being.

Common Nutritional Deficiencies That Impact Memory

Nutrition plays a crucial role in maintaining overall health, and it is especially important when it comes to memory and cognitive function. As caregivers of seniors with age-related memory decline, it is essential to understand the common nutritional deficiencies that can have a significant impact on their memory. By addressing these deficiencies, you can potentially improve their cognitive abilities and enhance their quality of life.

One common nutritional deficiency that affects memory is a lack of vitamin B12. This essential vitamin is responsible for maintaining healthy nerve cells and producing red blood cells. Studies have shown that low levels of vitamin B12 can lead to memory problems, confusion, and even dementia. Seniors are particularly at risk of vitamin B12 deficiency due to decreased absorption in the stomach. Including foods rich in vitamin B12, such as fish, meat, eggs, and dairy products, in their diet can help combat this deficiency.

Another vital nutrient for memory is omega-3 fatty acids. These healthy fats are essential for brain health and can improve memory and cognitive function. Unfortunately, seniors often have low levels of omega-3 fatty acids in their diet. Encourage them to consume fatty fish like salmon or mackerel, as well as walnuts, flaxseeds, and chia seeds, to boost their omega-3 intake.

Iron deficiency is another common nutritional deficiency that can impact memory. Iron is necessary for carrying oxygen to the brain, and inadequate levels can lead to cognitive impairment and poor memory. Include iron-rich foods like lean meats, beans, spinach, and fortified cereals in their meals to prevent iron deficiency.

Furthermore, inadequate levels of vitamin D can also contribute to memory problems. Vitamin D deficiency is prevalent among seniors, especially those who spend limited time outdoors. Encourage them to get some sunlight exposure and consume vitamin D-rich foods like fatty fish, fortified dairy products, and eggs to ensure they are meeting their vitamin D needs.

As caregivers, it is vital to be aware of these common nutritional deficiencies and take appropriate steps to address them. By ensuring that your seniors' diet is balanced and includes a variety of nutrient-rich foods, you can play a crucial role in supporting their memory and overall cognitive health. However, it is essential to consult with a healthcare professional or a registered dietitian before making any significant dietary changes or introducing supplements.

Dietary Recommendations for Improving Memory Function

Proper nutrition plays a crucial role in maintaining and improving memory function in seniors with age-related memory decline. As caregivers, it is important for you to understand the impact of diet on memory and provide the necessary support to enhance cognitive health. This subchapter will provide you with dietary recommendations that can effectively improve memory function in older adults.

1. Emphasize a Balanced Diet: Encourage a well-rounded diet that includes a variety of fruits, vegetables, whole grains, lean proteins, and healthy fats. This will provide the essential nutrients needed for optimal brain function. Include foods rich in antioxidants, such as berries, spinach, and nuts, to protect brain cells from damage.

2. Increase Omega-3 Fatty Acids: Omega-3 fatty acids, found in fatty fish like salmon, mackerel, and tuna, have been linked to improved memory function. Consider incorporating these

foods into the senior's diet or provide them with a high-quality omega-3 supplement.

3. Limit Sugar and Processed Foods: Excessive sugar intake and processed foods have been associated with memory impairment. Encourage the consumption of natural sugars found in fruits and limit the intake of sugary snacks, sodas, and processed foods.

4. Stay Hydrated: Dehydration can negatively impact cognitive function. Ensure that seniors are drinking enough water throughout the day. Consider including hydrating foods such as cucumbers, watermelon, and soups in their diet.

5. Maintain Vitamin B12 Levels: Low levels of vitamin B12 have been linked to memory decline. Encourage the consumption of foods rich in vitamin B12, such as eggs, dairy products, fish, and fortified cereals. In cases of deficiency, consult a healthcare professional for appropriate supplementation.

6. Incorporate Brain-Boosting Herbs and Spices: Certain herbs and spices have shown promising effects in improving memory function. Encourage the use of turmeric, rosemary, sage, and ginkgo biloba in cooking or as supplements. However, consult with a healthcare professional before introducing any new supplements.

7. Monitor Medications: Some medications can cause memory loss or cognitive impairment. Work closely with healthcare professionals to monitor medication side effects and explore alternative options if necessary.

Remember, dietary changes alone may not reverse memory decline, but they can contribute significantly to overall brain health. Combine these recommendations with other strategies such as memory training, cognitive exercises, and sleep optimization to provide comprehensive care for seniors with memory decline.

Chapter 9: Memory Loss and Sleep Disorders in Older Adults

The Relationship Between Sleep and Memory

Sleep plays a crucial role in memory consolidation, especially in older adults with age-related memory decline, dementia, Alzheimer's disease, or mild cognitive impairment. As caregivers, understanding the relationship between sleep and memory can help you provide better care for your seniors and implement effective memory loss prevention strategies.

During sleep, the brain undergoes a process called memory consolidation. This process helps transfer information from short-term memory to long-term memory, making it easier for seniors to retain and recall information. Lack of sleep or poor sleep quality can disrupt this process, leading to memory problems and cognitive decline.

In seniors, sleep disorders like insomnia, sleep apnea, or restless leg syndrome are common and can significantly impact memory. These sleep disorders often result in fragmented sleep, frequent awakenings, or difficulty falling asleep, leading to impaired memory functioning.

Furthermore, medications commonly prescribed to seniors, such as sedatives, antidepressants, or antihistamines, can interfere with sleep patterns and contribute to memory loss. It is important to consult with healthcare professionals to assess the potential side effects of medications and explore alternative options if necessary.

Nutritional deficiencies also play a role in memory loss. Certain vitamins and minerals, such as vitamin B12, vitamin D, and omega-3 fatty acids, are essential for brain health and proper sleep regulation. A well-balanced diet that includes these nutrients can improve sleep quality and enhance memory functioning.

As caregivers, you can support seniors in improving their sleep and memory by implementing a few strategies:

1. Establish a consistent sleep routine: Encourage seniors to go to bed and wake up at the same time every day to regulate their sleep-wake cycle.

2. Create a sleep-friendly environment: Ensure the bedroom is quiet, dark, and comfortable to promote quality sleep.

3. Encourage regular exercise: Physical activity during the day can promote better sleep at night and enhance memory functioning.

4. Limit caffeine and alcohol intake: Both substances can interfere with sleep patterns and should be consumed in moderation or avoided.

5. Promote relaxation techniques: Teach seniors relaxation techniques like deep breathing, meditation, or gentle stretching to help them unwind before bedtime.

Remember, caring for seniors with memory decline involves addressing various aspects of their well-being, including sleep. By understanding and implementing strategies to promote healthy sleep patterns, you can enhance their memory functioning and overall quality of life.

Sleep Disorders That Affect Memory in Seniors

As a caregiver for seniors with age-related memory decline, it is essential to understand the connection between sleep disorders and memory impairment. Sleep plays a crucial role in memory consolidation and overall brain health. When seniors struggle with sleep disorders, it can have a significant impact on their memory and cognitive function. In this subchapter, we will explore the various sleep disorders that can affect memory in seniors and provide strategies for caregivers to help manage and improve sleep quality.

One common sleep disorder among seniors is insomnia. Insomnia can make it challenging for seniors to fall asleep, stay asleep, or achieve restorative sleep. Research has shown that poor sleep quality and insomnia can lead to memory problems and cognitive decline. Caregivers can support seniors with insomnia by creating a calming bedtime routine, ensuring a comfortable sleep environment, and encouraging relaxation techniques such as deep breathing or meditation.

Another sleep disorder that affects memory in seniors is sleep apnea. Sleep apnea is characterized by interrupted breathing during sleep, leading to fragmented sleep and oxygen deprivation. This condition has been linked to memory impairment and an increased risk of developing dementia. Caregivers should be aware of the signs of sleep apnea, such as loud snoring, gasping for air during sleep, and excessive daytime sleepiness. Encouraging seniors to undergo a sleep study and providing them with appropriate treatment options, such as continuous positive airway pressure (CPAP) therapy, can greatly improve their sleep quality and memory function.

Restless legs syndrome (RLS) is another sleep disorder that affects memory in seniors. This neurological condition causes an irresistible urge to move the legs, often accompanied by uncomfortable sensations. RLS can lead to disrupted sleep and daytime fatigue, impacting memory and cognitive abilities. Caregivers can assist seniors with RLS by promoting a regular exercise routine, implementing relaxation techniques before bedtime, and discussing medication options with their healthcare provider.

Additionally, caregivers should be aware of the impact of medications and nutritional deficiencies on sleep and memory in seniors. Certain medications, such as sedatives or antidepressants, can interfere with sleep patterns and memory function. Nutritional deficiencies, particularly in vitamins B12 and D, have also been linked to sleep disturbances and memory problems. Collaborating with healthcare professionals to review medication regimens and ensuring seniors have a well-balanced diet can help improve sleep quality and memory function.

In conclusion, sleep disorders can significantly affect memory in seniors with age-related memory decline. As caregivers, it is crucial to recognize the signs of sleep disorders and implement strategies to improve sleep quality. By addressing sleep issues and promoting healthy sleep habits, caregivers can support seniors in maintaining optimal memory function and overall well-being.

Promoting Healthy Sleep Habits for Memory Enhancement

Introduction:

As caregivers of seniors with age-related memory decline, it is important to understand how sleep habits can impact memory function. Sleep plays a crucial role in memory consolidation and overall cognitive health. In this subchapter, we will explore the significance of healthy sleep habits in memory enhancement and provide practical strategies for caregivers to promote better sleep for their loved ones.

The Importance of Sleep for Memory:

Sleep is a complex process that allows our brains to consolidate and store information gathered throughout the day. For seniors with age-related memory decline, ensuring they get enough quality sleep is vital for memory enhancement. Research has shown that a lack of sleep can impair memory formation, increase forgetfulness, and even contribute to the progression of conditions like dementia and Alzheimer's disease.

Strategies for Promoting Healthy Sleep Habits:

1. Establish a Consistent Sleep Routine: Help your loved one establish a regular sleep schedule by setting fixed bedtimes and wake-up times. Consistency is key to regulating their internal body clock and promoting better sleep quality.

2. Create a Restful Environment: Ensure the sleeping area is quiet, dark, and comfortable. Use blackout curtains, earplugs, or white noise machines to minimize disturbances. Also, consider

investing in a supportive mattress and pillows to enhance comfort.

3. Encourage Relaxation Techniques: Help your loved one wind down before bedtime by engaging in relaxing activities such as reading, listening to calming music, or practicing gentle stretching exercises. Avoid stimulating activities or electronics close to bedtime.

4. Limit Stimulants: Advise your loved one to avoid caffeine, nicotine, and alcohol, especially in the hours leading up to bedtime. These substances can disrupt sleep patterns and hinder memory consolidation.

5. Promote Physical Activity: Encourage regular exercise during the day, as it can improve sleep quality. However, advise against vigorous workouts close to bedtime, as they may have the opposite effect.

6. Monitor Medications: Some medications can interfere with sleep quality. Consult with a healthcare professional to ensure that your loved one's medications are not causing sleep disturbances and discuss possible alternatives if necessary.

Conclusion:

By prioritizing healthy sleep habits, caregivers can significantly enhance memory function in seniors with age-related memory decline. Remember that promoting better sleep is a multifaceted approach that involves establishing a consistent routine, creating a restful environment, encouraging relaxation techniques, limiting stimulants, promoting physical activity, and monitoring medications. By implementing these strategies, caregivers can play a crucial role in supporting their loved ones' cognitive health and overall well-being.

Chapter 10: Memory Loss in Seniors: Coping Strategies for Caregivers

Emotional Support for Caregivers of Seniors with Memory Loss

Caring for a senior with memory loss can be an emotionally challenging journey. As a caregiver, it is essential to prioritize your emotional well-being as you navigate the complexities of age-related memory decline, dementia, Alzheimer's disease, or mild cognitive impairment. In this subchapter, we will explore the importance of emotional support for caregivers and provide practical strategies to help you cope with the unique challenges you may face.

First and foremost, it is crucial to acknowledge and validate your feelings. It is normal to experience a range of emotions, including frustration, sadness, and even guilt. Remember that your emotions are valid, and seeking support from others who understand your situation can be tremendously helpful. Connect with support groups, either in person or online, where you can share your experiences, gain insight from others, and find solace in knowing you are not alone.

Self-care is equally important. Taking care of your own physical and emotional needs is not selfish but necessary for your well-being. Make time for activities that bring you joy and relaxation, whether it's reading a book, going for a walk, or enjoying a hobby. Prioritize regular exercise, eat a balanced diet, and ensure you get enough restful sleep. By caring for yourself, you will have more energy and resilience to care for your loved one.

Seeking professional help can also be beneficial. Consider consulting a therapist or counselor who specializes in caregiving or geriatric care. They can provide a safe space for you to express your feelings, offer guidance on effective coping strategies, and help you develop healthy boundaries.

Additionally, it is essential to educate yourself about memory loss and its associated conditions. Understanding the progression of the disease, available treatments, and management strategies can help you feel more empowered and confident in your caregiving role. Educate yourself through reputable sources, attend workshops or webinars, and consult healthcare professionals for accurate information.

Finally, remember to celebrate small victories and find moments of joy amidst the challenges. Cherish the meaningful connections you can still have with your loved one, even if their memory is impaired. Engage in activities that stimulate their cognitive abilities, such as memory games or reminiscence therapy. Create a supportive environment filled with familiar objects, photographs, and music that can trigger positive memories.

Caregiving for a senior with memory loss is undoubtedly a challenging journey, but with the right emotional support and self-care strategies, it can also be a deeply rewarding experience. Remember, you are not alone, and by prioritizing your emotional well-being, you can provide the best care for your loved one while maintaining your own mental and emotional health.

Practical Tips for Enhancing Memory Support

As a caregiver of a senior with age-related memory decline, it is essential to equip yourself with practical strategies to enhance memory support. These tips will not only help your loved one maintain their cognitive abilities but also improve their overall quality of life. Here are some practical tips for enhancing memory support:

1. Establish a Routine: Seniors with memory decline benefit from a structured daily routine. Consistency helps them feel more secure and reduces confusion. Ensure that daily activities such as meals, medication, and exercise occur at the same time each day.

2. Use Memory Aids: Memory aids, such as calendars, pill organizers, and reminder apps, can be invaluable tools for seniors with memory impairment. Encourage your loved one to use these aids to help them remember important dates, appointments, and tasks.

3. Simplify the Environment: Minimize distractions and clutter in your loved one's living space. Create a calm and organized environment that promotes focus and reduces cognitive overload. Label drawers and cabinets to help them find items easily.

4. Encourage Physical Exercise: Regular physical exercise has been shown to improve memory and cognitive function.

Encourage your loved one to engage in activities such as walking, swimming, or yoga. Physical activity increases blood flow to the brain, promoting brain health.

5. Stimulate the Mind: Engage your loved one in activities that stimulate their cognitive abilities. Puzzles, word games, reading, and learning new skills can help maintain memory function. Consider enrolling them in memory training programs or cognitive exercises specifically designed for seniors.

6. Ensure Adequate Nutrition: Nutritional deficiencies can contribute to memory decline in seniors. Ensure that your loved one follows a balanced diet rich in fruits, vegetables, whole grains, and omega-3 fatty acids. Consult a healthcare professional to determine if any supplements are necessary.

7. Promote Quality Sleep: Sleep plays a crucial role in memory consolidation. Help your loved one establish a regular sleep schedule and create a relaxing bedtime routine. Minimize daytime napping to avoid disrupting nighttime sleep.

8. Communicate Effectively: When interacting with your loved one, use clear and concise language. Break down complex tasks into smaller, manageable steps. Give them ample time to process information and avoid rushing or pressuring them.

9. Seek Support: Caring for a senior with memory decline can be challenging. Connect with support groups or organizations specializing in memory loss to access resources, share experiences, and learn coping strategies from fellow caregivers.

Remember, every individual is unique, and what works for one person may not work for another. Be patient, compassionate, and flexible in your approach. By implementing these practical tips, you can provide the best possible memory support for your loved one and improve their overall well-being.

Seeking Professional Help and Resources for Caregivers

As a caregiver for a senior with age-related memory decline, dementia, Alzheimer's disease, or any other form of memory impairment, it is essential to recognize the importance of seeking professional help and utilizing available resources. This subchapter aims to provide caregivers like you with valuable information on how to access the support and assistance you need to navigate through this challenging journey.

Professional help is crucial in understanding the specific condition your loved one is facing and developing effective care strategies. One of the first steps you should take is to consult with a healthcare professional specializing in geriatric care or memory disorders. They can conduct a comprehensive assessment, diagnose the condition, and provide guidance on appropriate treatment options.

In addition to medical professionals, there are various resources available to caregivers that can offer support and knowledge. Support groups specifically designed for caregivers of seniors with memory decline can provide a safe space to share experiences, exchange advice, and find emotional support. These groups can be found in local community centers, hospitals, or online platforms.

Furthermore, caregiver support organizations and associations offer a wealth of information on memory care, coping strategies, and available resources. They often provide educational workshops, training programs, and access to experts in the field. Joining these organizations can connect you with a network of individuals who understand the challenges you face and can offer guidance.

Depending on your loved one's specific needs, you may also benefit from seeking the help of professional caregivers or home care services. These individuals are trained to provide specialized care, assistance with activities of daily living, and ensure the safety and well-being of your loved one. They can offer respite for you as a caregiver, allowing you to take breaks and prioritize your own self-care.

Additionally, it is crucial to explore memory loss prevention strategies, memory training, and cognitive exercises for your loved one. This could involve working with a cognitive therapist or participating in memory enhancement programs specifically designed for seniors with memory decline.

Remember, seeking professional help and utilizing available resources is not a sign of weakness but rather a testament to your dedication as a caregiver. By accessing these resources, you are equipping yourself with the knowledge and support needed to provide the best possible care for your loved one.

www.ingramcontent.com/pod-product-compliance
Lightning Source LLC
Chambersburg PA
CBHW021751150726
47989CB00004B/1612